HEALTH BENEFITS OF AVOCADO

For Cooking and Health

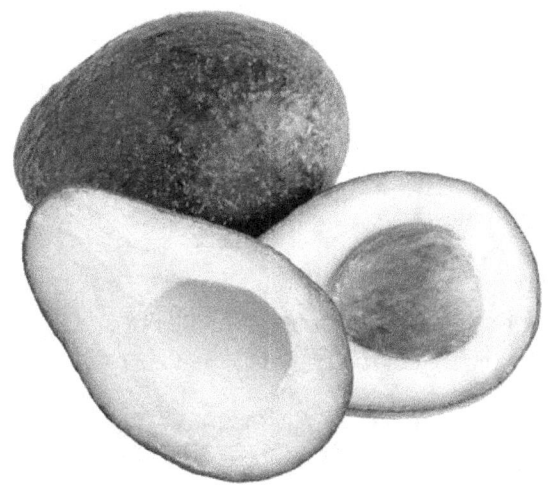

Health Learning Series

M. Usman

Mendon Cottage Books

JD-Biz Publishing

Disclaimer

The information is this book is provided for informational purposes only. It is not intended to be used and medical advice or a substitute for proper medical treatment by a qualified health care provider. The information is believed to be accurate as presented based on research by the author.

The contents have not been evaluated by the U.S. Food and Drug Administration or any other Government or Health Organization and the contents in this book are not to be used to treat cure or prevent disease.

The author or publisher is not responsible for the use or safety of any diet, procedure or treatment mentioned in this book. The author or publisher is not responsible for errors or omissions that may exist.

Warning

The Book is for informational purposes only and before taking on any diet, treatment or medical procedure, it is recommended to consult with your primary health care provider.

Check out some of the other Healthy Gardening Series books at Amazon.com

Gardening Series on Amazon

Check out some of the other Health Learning Series books at Amazon.com

Health Learning Series on Amazon

Table of Contents

Introduction

Health Benefits of Avocado

The Pear Shaped Fruit

You might have heard the name "Avocado" a thousand times and wonder what it is. Well for starters, avocado is a fruit that is pear shaped in appearance. If you're into fruits and veggies and believe in natural ways of living an ailment free life, then this book is all you need. Even if you don't like fruits, you should still know about this one. Being a nutritionist, I would crown this fruit as the "king of all fruits" because of its nutritional value and health benefits. The interesting thing is that all these benefits come with no side effects, which are quite frequent with the advertised pills and supplements.

In our daily life we give value to things that are ready to eat or things that we can eat on the go. No wonder diseases like heart attack, high blood pressure, arthritis and obesity are so common in western lifestyle. Yes, I called obesity a disease. To you obesity might only mean having socially unacceptable outlook, but medicine people would tell you that obesity is the harbinger of countless diseases. The cure and control of all these things comes with one single fruit. Yes, you guessed it right. It's avocado that promises you not only a healthy outlook but also a healthy inside too. Above all, the taste of this fruit is something that would surely tickle your taste buds.

This book has been divided into four sections. The first section will inform you about avocado and tell you what it is, its history and its nutritional value. The second section of the book is about the health benefits of avocado. Different diseases that can be cured with the help of avocado have also been mentioned. The role of avocado in weight loss and nourishing of skin and hair has also been discussed. The third section lists some golden tips related to this fruit. The final section is left for conclusion.

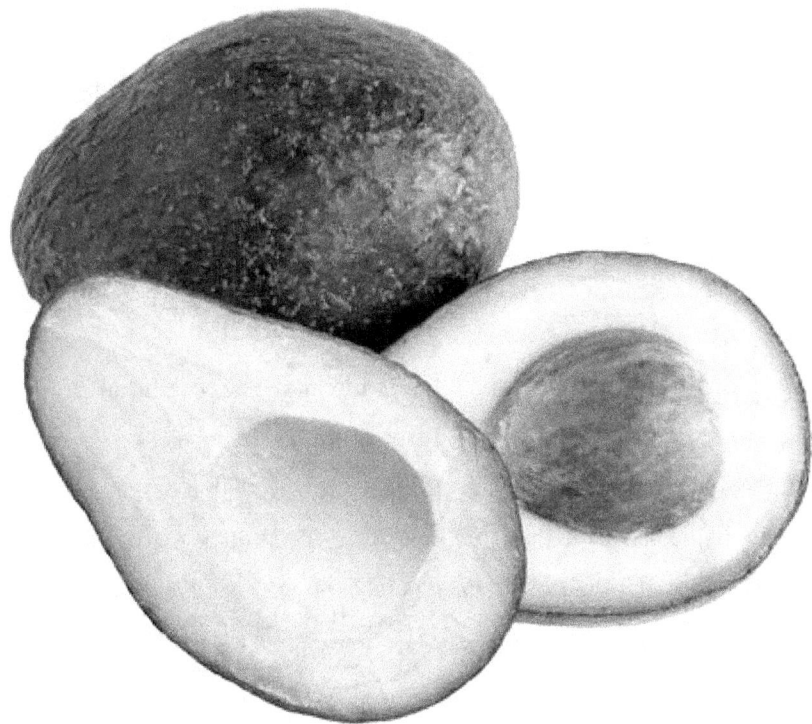

Section 1: Avocado

Chapter 1: What is Avocado?

Avocado

Avocado is a tree native to Mexico and Central America. It is classified in the family of the flowering plant family *Lauraceae* along with camphor and cinnamon. This fruit is mainly cultivated in the tropical regions. However, sometimes it is also suitable for growth in more temperate regions. It can also be found in Mediterranean regions.

Avocado Tree

The Avocado tree is erect, usually 30 feet in length. The length can, however, vary up to 60 feet or more. Its trunk is 12-24 inches in diameter or sometimes smaller than that. Its leaves are evergreen with a dark green color on the upper side and whitish on the inner side. The tree bears pale green or yellow green flowers; the flowers lack petals and have 9 stamens and two orange nectar glands.

Avocado Fruit

The fruit is oval shaped and can technically be classified as the member of berries. You can consider the fruit as nearly round. It may vary from 3 to 13 inches long and is up to 6 inches wide. The skin may be dark green, reddish purple, dark purple, deep green or yellow green. Tiny yellow dots are present on the skin that may either be smooth or pebbled. Some fruits bear bright green flesh beneath their skin, however, generally the skin is pale to rich yellow in color. The fruit has a buttery or nutlike flavor.

Chapter 2: History of Avocado

It is believed that avocados originated from the state of Mexico. There is evidence that they have been utilized by the Mexicans for almost 10,000 years. These fruits were first discovered by the Spanish Conquistadors. However, some fossil evidence shows that a species, similar to avocados but more widespread, was present as far as Northern California.

Avocado fruit was first mentioned by Martin Fernandez de Enciso in 1519, when he wrote a published account on these fruits. After this, the popularity of the fruit began to grow. During the 1700s, the Europeans used Avocados as a spread for biscuits. These trees were introduced in California in 1856 and in Florida in 1850. They arrived in Indonesia in 1750, in Brazil in 1809, in Israel in 1908 and in South Africa and Australia in the later part of the nineteenth century.

Chapter 3: How to Choose the Right Avocado

Choosing the right avocado can be a challenging task, especially for those who don't buy fruits often. Furthermore, there are many varieties of avocados in the market, and that makes it difficult to choose the right avocado. For buying a good avocado, it is essential to know about the properties of each variety. You need to look for signs like the taste and the ripeness of the fruit. Some tips for choosing a good avocado are as follows:

- There are two major producers of Avocado in the United States. The products offered in a store might differ depending upon the geographical location and the season. The first type of avocado is the California avocados. These avocados are available around the year. The most common variety of these avocados is the Hass avocado. It has a rough bumpy skin and a rich flavor. The other type of avocado are the Florida avocados, which are also rich bumpy avocados available for 8 months from July to February. They are twice the size of the California avocados.

- You need to determine the purpose of choosing the fruit. If you need the fruit on an immediate basis, you would want ready to eat, ripe avocados. However if you don't need them for immediate purposes, you can purchase the avocado and then ripen it at home.

- The third phase is checking the fruit. For this purpose, hold the fruit in the palm of your hand. Gently squeeze the fruit. Be careful not to press the fruit with your finger-tips as it can lead to bruising. The fruit, which is ripe, will be soft and will easily yield to pressure. The ripe fruit can be eaten. However, if the fruit is hard, it won't yield to the pressure easily . This fruit isn't suitable for eating, yet. However if you don't need the fruit on immediate basis, you can take the fruit home and then ripen it.

- Choose the avocado that has a ripe skin as avocados not shiny enough aren't suitable for eating.

- Avoid avocados that are too soft. Too much softness in the fruit indicates that the fruit is too ripe to eat.

You need to know here that you can't master the art of choosing the right avocado in a day or two. Like everything else, you need more practice. After buying avocados for ten to twelve times, you will be an expert in choosing the right ones.

Chapter 4: Nutritional Breakdown of Avocados

Avocado is a nutrient dense food loaded with minerals, vitamins, carbohydrates and few other calories. One fifth of a medium avocado contains 50 calories and has approximately 20 vitamins and minerals (now you know why we called it nutrient dense).

The following few tables will provide you with the nutritional breakdown of avocados.

Amount per 1 cup, cubes

Amount of Carbohydrates:

Total carbohydrate	12.8g
Starch	0.2g
Sugars	0.1g
Dietary Fiber	10.1g

Amount of Fats:

Total fat	22.0g
Saturated fat	3.2g
Mon saturated fat	14.7g
Polyunsaturated fat	2.7g
Total trans-polyenic fatty acids	N.A
Total trans-moenic fatty acids	N.A
Total omega 6 fatty acids	2534g
Total omega 3 fatty acids	165g

Amount of Proteins:

Protein	3.0g

Minerals:

Calcium	18g
Iron	0.8g
Magnesium	43.5g
Zinc	1.0g
Sodium	10.5g
Phosphorus	78.0g
Manganese	0.2g
Fluoride	10.5mcg
Selenium	0.6mcg

Vitamins:

Vitamin C	15g
Vitamin A	219 IU
Vitamin D	N.A
Thiamine	0.1g
Vitamin B6	0.4g
Folate	122mcg
Vitamin B12	0.0mcg
Vitamin K	31.7mcg
Niacin	2.6 mg

Amount of Sterols:

Cholesterol	0.0mg
Polysterols	N.A

Other Constituents:

Water	11.0g
Ash	2.4g
Caffeine	0.0g

Theobromine	0.0g
Alcohol	0.0g

Section 2: Health Benefits of Avocados

The previous section of the book gave you a basic introduction about avocados like: what it is, its history, how to choose the right avocado and its nutritional breakdown. This section will inform you about what is so special about this fruit that makes it unique among the large variety of the fruits available in the market. The thing that makes this fruit unique is its large number of benefits. This section will cover such benefits. This section has been divided into three chapters. The first chapter will list some diseases that can be cured with the help of avocados. In the second chapter, avocado benefits for weight loss have been discussed whereas in the last chapter some benefits of avocado relating to skin and hair have been discussed.

Chapter 5: Protection against diseases

Avocado is quite beneficial against a bunch of diseases ranging from cardiovascular diseases to diabetes and raised cholesterol levels in the body. Some benefits of avocado against different diseases, as proved through scientific studies, are given below:

1. Cardio vascular health.

Avocados are highly beneficial for cardiovascular diseases. This benefit is on the top of your list because cardiovascular diseases like heart attack and stroke are still the leading cause of death in America.

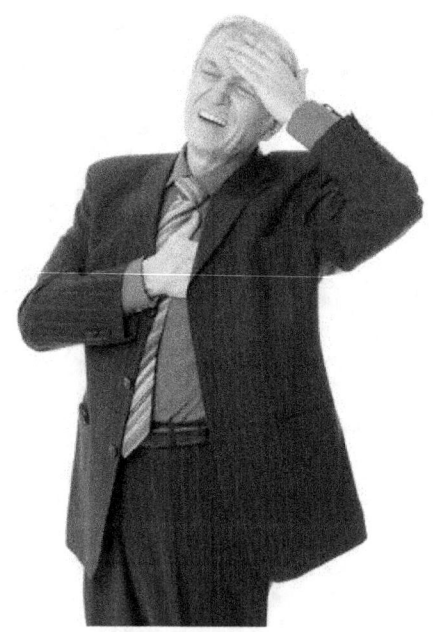

According to the experts, increased use of processed food and eating a diet rich in saturated fats is the essential risk factor for causing cardiovascular diseases. The advice here is to lower the intake of saturated fats and increase the amount of unsaturated fatty acids in the diet. Here comes the role of avocados. This fruit is a rich source of monosaturted oleic acid. A recent research held in America has revealed that the use of avocados can reduce the level of "bad cholesterol" (low-density lipoprotein (LDL)) while at the same time increase the amount of "good cholesterol" (high density lipoprotein (HDL)). Other than this, avocados also contain large amounts of vitamin E in them, which helps in the prevention of oxidation and production of free radicals. In other words, avocado is a natural anti-oxidant. It also contains folate that reduces the dangerous homocystiene levels in the blood.

2. Lowering of cholesterol.

Avocado oil is quite beneficial for controlling high cholesterol levels in the body. Avocados contain monosaturated oil, known as the oleic acid, which helps in lowering the overall cholesterol levels in the body. In a study, it was proved that patients with high cholesterol levels who ate avocado fruits showed a significant improvement in their cholesterol status. So if your doctor has diagnosed you with high cholesterol and has advised you to eat cholesterol lowering food then there can't be anything as useful as eating avocados.

3. Regulation of Blood Pressure.

Avocados contain potassium in them that is helpful in regulating blood pressure in the body. Once your blood pressure gets back to normal, you're less likely to get other diseases like heart attack, stroke and kidney disease.

4. A heart booster.

Vitamin B6 present in avocados helps in the regulation of homocysteine levels. High levels of homocysteine can lead to an increased risk of heart diseases. Other than vitamin B6, avocado contains glutathione and mono saturated fats that are also helpful in the maintenance of a healthy heart.

5. Anti-Inflammatory Properties.

Avocados contain polyhydroxylated fatty alcohols (PFAS). PFAS are present mostly in sea weeds and other plants and are extremely rare in land plants. This makes avocado a very unusual fruit. The PFAS, polysterols and flavonoids present in avocados, provide the body with different anti-inflammatory properties that help in fighting against a variety of diseases. These compounds put a stop to the synthesis of prostaglandins, main culprits of inflammation. This way avocados shield your body from inflammation and all the damage done by it.

6. Protection of Eye.

Avocados contain carotenoids that protect the eye against cataracts and macular degeneration.

7. Fights cancer.

Another important health benefit of avocado is its ability to prevent the growth of cancer in the body and the support given to the body's natural defense mechanisms. Avocados contain a combination of cancer fighters such as vitamin E, Lutein, carotenoids, oleic acid and glutathione.

Research has shown that avocados are natural protectors against breast cancer as they contain a concentrated amount of carotenoids and oleic acid. Another research has shown that women with increased leutin in their diet are at a lower risk of breast cancer. Yet another laboratory study published in the *Journal Of Nutritional Biochemistry* has shown that an extract of avocado containing tocopherols and carotenoids is quite helpful in stopping and minimizing the growth of androgen dependent and androgen independent prostate cancer cells.

Avocados are a rich source of vitamin E succinate, which is helpful in reducing the risk of cancer of the breast and prostate. Research has shown that vitamin E can turn off many different agents of cancer cells and stop their reproduction. This slows down the ability of the cancer cells to replicate. Other than this, vitamin E has also shown its ability to stimulate the cancer cells to undergo apoptosis which, in simple terms, is also known as "cell suicide".

8. Anti-ageing properties.

As avocados are rich in anti-oxidants, they help in the prevention of ageing symptoms. Glutathione, present in avocados, boosts the immune system of the body that slows the aging process in the body and helps in generating a healthy nervous system.

9. Diabetes.

In 2012, nearly 3,000,000 people in U.S and the U.K were diagnosed with diabetes. If this rate continues, 5 million people will have diabetes at the end of 2025, putting a huge pressure on hospitals to treat people.

The most common symptom of diabetes is a sudden increase in thirst and hunger and frequent urination. Unexplained weight loss and vision problems are among other symptoms. So if you are experiencing these symptoms, it's best to inform your doctor. Other than visiting the doctor, you can eat avocados too. The oleic acid present in them is popular for its ability to lower the bad cholesterol while at the same time raising the good cholesterol in the body; keeping the cholesterol levels in check is quite vital for people with diabetes. Moreover, more monosaturated acid present in the diet is also beneficial for reducing triglyceride levels in the body which helps the insulin function and blood glucose level in the body. High fiber content of avocado is also very essential in regulating blood sugar.

10. Arthritis.

Osteoarthritis is quite a painful disease affecting millions of people every year in the UK and U.S. The symptoms of this disease include things like pain in the back and stiffness and soreness in the joints. Many foods like sugar, milk, red meat and wheat can worsen these symptoms. However avocado is reported to reduce the pain of arthritis as it contains a large amount of monosaturated fats, antioxidants like vitamin E and C, phytosterols and a variety of carotenoids that help in reducing the inflammation causing arthritis.

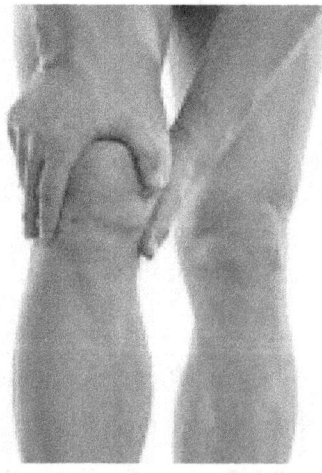

11. Increase in nutrient absorption.

Avocados speed up the absorption of nutrients from your gut. Not only is it rich in nutrients itself but it also boosts other nutrients that you might eat. A study showed that when participants ate salads, in which avocados were included, they absorbed five times the amount of carotenoids as compared to those who didn't include avocados in salads. The increase in the nutrient absorption helps in fending off different diseases.

12. Prevention of Birth Defects.

Avocados are helpful in preventing birth defects. They are rich in folate, a vitamin B commonly known as folic acid. A cup of avocados provide 23% of daily value of folate. This high amount helps in the prevention of birth defects such as spina bifida, neural tube defect, alcohol related birth defects, cleft lip, fetal alcohol syndrome and microcephaly.

13. Helps Against Eczema.

Another benefit of avocado fruit is that it helps against eczema. For those of you who don't know about this disease, eczema is a medical condition in which skin patches become rough and inflamed that causes itching and in some cases, bleeding in the body. Sometimes it can even cause irritation in the whole body. However this disease has no apparent cause. Avocado oil helps relieve people from eczema as it contains fat soluble vitamins like A, D, K and E that help in the maintenance of a healthy skin. So if you are suffering from eczema, apply avocado oil in the parts that cause irritation and produce an itchy sensation.

Chapter 6: Avocados for Weight Loss

There is a long disproven fact, yet still persistent belief among some people, that eating food makes us fat. The more we eat, the fatter we get. But it's not just about how much you eat. What you eat also matters a lot. The more you fill your plate with sugars and saturated fats, the more you're likely to gain weight.

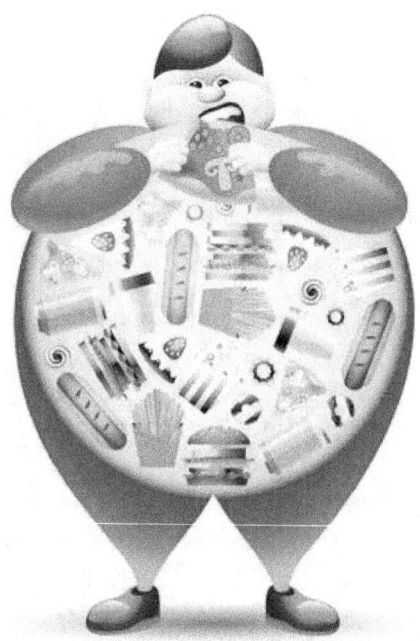

There is much debate in the world whether saturated fatty acids are really harmful for the health or not. However, a far worse culprit than saturated fats has been found and it is the trans and hydrogenated fats found in foods like margarine and treated vegetable oil. There is also evidence that the massive increase in refined carbohydrates is an effective weight gain trigger.

Avocados contain monounsaturated fats in them which help aid in weight loss. 100 gm of avocados provide 160 calories, while this might sound like a lot to you, these calories comes from a healthy source i.e. monosaturated fatty acids. In avocados, more than two thirds of calories come from monounsaturated oleic acid. Some studies have indicated that the monounsaturated oleic acid is more beneficial to the body as a slow burning energy source as compared to saturated fats. Moreover, increasing the intake of monounsaturated acid decreases the level of saturated fats and carbohydrates. All this results in better weight control; remarkable improvement in the glycemic control and improved insulin sensitivity.

According to a research published in the Nutrition Journal, eating one half of an avocado daily may satisfy a person's hunger needs. For this study, the researchers chose 26 healthy and overweight individuals. The participants were required to eat normal food over five sessions. Three lunches were included in a day. In the first lunch, there was no avocado included whereas in the second and third lunches avocado was included. It was found that participants ate less in those meals that included avocados in them. Higher content of fiber in avocados is responsible for this hunger satisfying effect.

Apart from helping in weight loss, the way avocados increase nutrient absorption in the diet can help in reducing hunger. This is because feeling hunger is, in most cases, not associated with our bodies need for more food but with many other factors. One of these factors is that people don't drink enough water during the day time and mistake their thirst for hunger. So the next time you feel hungry, try drinking a glass of water instead of gulping snacks. Another factor that contributes to feeling of hunger is that your body doesn't get enough nutrients in the previous meals which is depicted in the form of hunger. By eating foods like avocados, you are less likely to feel hungry. This is due to the contents present in avocado.

Chapter 7: Avocados for Skin and Hair:

Avocados are quite beneficial for skin and hair growth too. Now you might be wondering what is so special in avocados that make them beneficial for hair and skin? This chapter will answer this question.

Avocados for Skin

Avocados contain healthy fatty acids, vitamins and anti-oxidants in them that nourish your skin from the inside. Avocados are also a great source of anti-oxidant carotenoids like beta carotene, alpha carotene, zexanthin and leutin. These ingredients provide significant protection to the skin from the damage inflicted by free radicals. Research has supported the fact that high amounts of carotenoids in the diet can improve the skin's thickness, tone and general appearance.

Other than carotenoids, avocados also contain Vitamin C in them. A good amount of vitamin C is quite beneficial for healthy skin, as it contains strong anti-oxidant potential. Vitamin C is also needed by the body for the creation of elastin and collagen, which binds the skin cells together and helps in maintaining the firmness of skin.

Yet another skin oxidant present in avocado is vitamin E. It helps in preventing the free radical damage by oxidizing the fats present in the skin that lead to aging. Moreover it also helps in reducing rashes on the skin by removing the toxins that lead to premature ageing. Other than this, it also helps in eliminating wrinkles and gives the skin a youthful glow. Research studies have shown that vitamin E helps in the reduction of effects UVB and UVA radiations from the exposure to sun.

Avocados contain high amounts of oleic acid in them that is beneficial for the skin. This monounsaturated fatty acid maintains moisture in the upper layer of the skin. Moreover, it is helpful in regenerating damaged skin and reduces facial irritation and redness.

How to use

For applying avocados on the skin, the general method used is the avocado and honey skin treatment. For this method, you would need ½ peeled avocado, 1 tablespoon sugar, lemon juice and two tablespoons of honey. First of all, wash your face with warm water. After that, mash the avocado and mix it with the above mentioned ingredients. Now, apply the paste gently on the skin until the face and a bit of neck portion is covered. Leave the mask on for 15 minutes then wash it with warm water. After this process, notice the glow in your skin. You can also use this paste anywhere on your body. Using the same method, leave the mask on the whole body for approximately 15 minutes and after that, take a shower or bath in lukewarm water.

Avocados for Hair

The monounsaturated fatty acid content that is high in avocados accounts for its benefits for hair. Many people have dry, damaged hair that become weak because of poor nutrition, chemical treatments and environmental pollution. When the monounsaturated fats are applied in the form of a hair mask, they can nourish, moisturize and strengthen the hair strands, thus improving the way the hair looks and protecting it from further damage. Applying avocado oil on the hair stimulates blood flow in the hair follicles. In this way you end up having stronger and healthier hair.

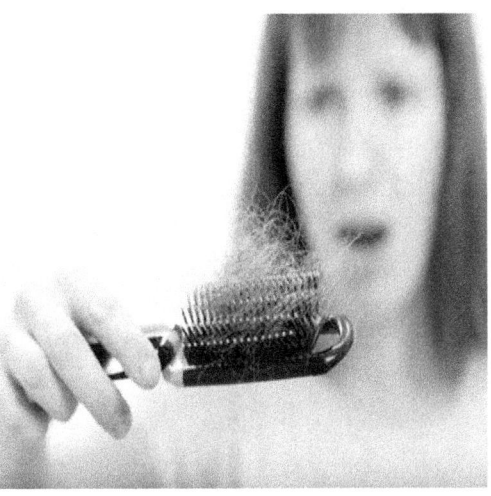

Avocado also contains phytosterols, monounsaturated fatty acids and vitamin E, all of which are quite beneficial for the hair. They absorb into the scalp and hair shafts. This not only is highly protective against the environmental stress and damage, it also stimulates new hair growth and follicles. In a crux, the combination of different contents present in avocado have a quite beneficial combined effect and help in hair growth.

How to use?

For applying avocado on your hair, the general method used is the avocado, butter and eggs hair treatment. For this method, combine butter and egg yolk and mix them well together. After that mash the avocado and add it to egg yolk and butter. Now wash your hair. After that, apply the mixture on your hair and leave it for about 1-2 hours. After two hours, wash your hair thoroughly. After this whole process, your hair will shine and become smooth.Another method for applying avocado to your hair is by the hot avocado oil treatment. For this method you would need 1 tablespoon of olive oil, 1 tablespoon of avocado oil and 1 soft and clean towel. First of all, mix avocado and olive oil in a small pot and heat them gently on low flame until they are slightly warm. Now, massage the mixture in a circular motion on your hair. Leave on your hair for fifteen minutes. Now soak the hair in warm water and take it out. Wrap a towel around your hair and keep it on for about 10 minutes. Finally, take off the towel and shampoo and condition your hair.

Section 3: Including Avocado In daily diet
Chapter 8: Recipes for Avocado

Some recipes that include avocado are mentioned here.

Avocado and Egg Break Fast Pizza.

For making this recipe, take a pizza and top it with avocado and an egg mashed in any style. You can also add some extra vegetables to add more flavor to the pizza.

Avocado Buckwheat Pancake.

For this recipe, top avocado on pancakes. By adding avocado to the recipe, you won't need to add any oil or butter.

Lemon Avocado Juice.

For making this juice, blend 1 glass of water, cucumber, ginger, avocado and greens (such as spinach) together and enjoy the drink.

Avocado Watermelon Salad.

You can also present avocado as a salad. Not only is this salad nutritious, it looks delicious too. You can make this salad my mixing watermelon, radish and avocado topped with mint.

Avocado with Tuna.

This is another recipe quite beneficial for health. To make it, mash avocado with a can of tuna and season it with pepper, salt and other herbs as you like.

Avocado Lettuce and Tomato Sandwich

The ingredients for this recipe include fat free mayonnaise, romaine lettuce, whole grain bread, Swiss cheese and cucumber. For making this recipe, add all these ingredients into a sandwich. The heart healthy fats will fill you up quickly and you won't need another snack for some hours.

Raw Avocado Soup.

This is a summer recipe. The ingredients of this recipe include fresh green peas, cucumber, avocado and mint. Tahini and lemon can also be added to add more flavor.

Sunday Smoothie: Avocado and Banana.

The ingredients for this dish are 1chopped avocado, 2 tablespoon honey and 1 cup sweet yogurt. To make the recipe, mix all the ingredients well in a glass and enjoy your Sunday with this Sunday Smoothie.

Black Bean Mushroom and Avocado Breakfast Scramble.

This dish makes a hearty protein packed vegetarian breakfast. The ingredients of this dish include 2 tablespoon olive oil, 1 small clove garlic, ½ small avocado, a few cilantro leaves and 1 cup white buttoned mushrooms. First of all add olive oil in a pot and heat it on a medium flame. Now add onions and mushrooms while constantly stirring it for 5 minutes. Now add eggs in them and stir constantly until the mixture is totally cooked. Taste and add additional salt if you like. Now top it with avocado and cilantro leaves. The dish is now ready to eat.

Spooky Avocado Witchy Finger.

The ingredients of this recipe include 4 avocados, 1 tablespoon lemon juice, 2 ounces of goat cheese, 1 tablespoon chilli pepper, 1 tablespoon chilli powder and 1 ounce prosciutto slices. First of all, cut each avocado into slices. Now place them in medium bowl and gently toss them in lemon juice. Now fill the centre of each avocado with goat cheese. Sprinkle it with salt and pepper and wrap each avocado with 1/3 slices of prosciutto until cheese is secured. Now the dish is ready to eat.

This section has informed you about some recipes including avocado. In conclusion, although avocado can be eaten raw, you need to try out these recipes to add a little more fun in your diet.

Section 4: Fun Facts about Avocado

The previous section mentioned some recipes including avocado. This section will inform you about some fun facts about avocado. Some fun facts about this pear shaped fruit are given below:

- Avocados are a fruit and not a vegetable and belong to the genus Persea in the Lauraceae family.
- Avocados are baby friendly. They are a good snack to feed to babies.
- Avocados are one of the unique foods that contain heart-healthy monounsaturated fats that help in boosting good cholesterol and lowering bad cholesterol in the body.
- In Brazil, avocados are mixed with ice cream to make dessert.
- California produces about 90% of the whole avocado crop in America.
- Avocados are also known as alligator pear because of their shape, green texture and rough skin.
- Consumption of avocados is increasing on a daily basis due to the large number of benefits associated with it. For an estimation, 1.6 billion avocados were consumed in the United States during 2012.
- Avocados mature on the tree but they ripen once they are off the tree.
- 43% of all U.S. households buy avocados.
- A single California tree can produce up to 500 avocados in a year.

Section 5: Conclusion

Now here comes the end of the book. By now you must have completely known and understood why I called avocados "the king of fruits". The list of health benefits of this fruit is endless and there are endless ways you can use this fruit. Things can't get easier than this, right? All you need to do is add avocados in your meals, soups or salads and see the ailments wither away. Eating avocados on daily basis is a complete weight loss plan on its own and if you make a habit of eating this fruit, you won't put on any more pounds- I can guarantee this much. All the benefits mentioned here make avocados among the top most beneficial fruits in the world. So what are you waiting for? Do buy avocados next time you buy groceries.

Check out some of the other JD-Biz Publishing books

Gardening Series on Amazon

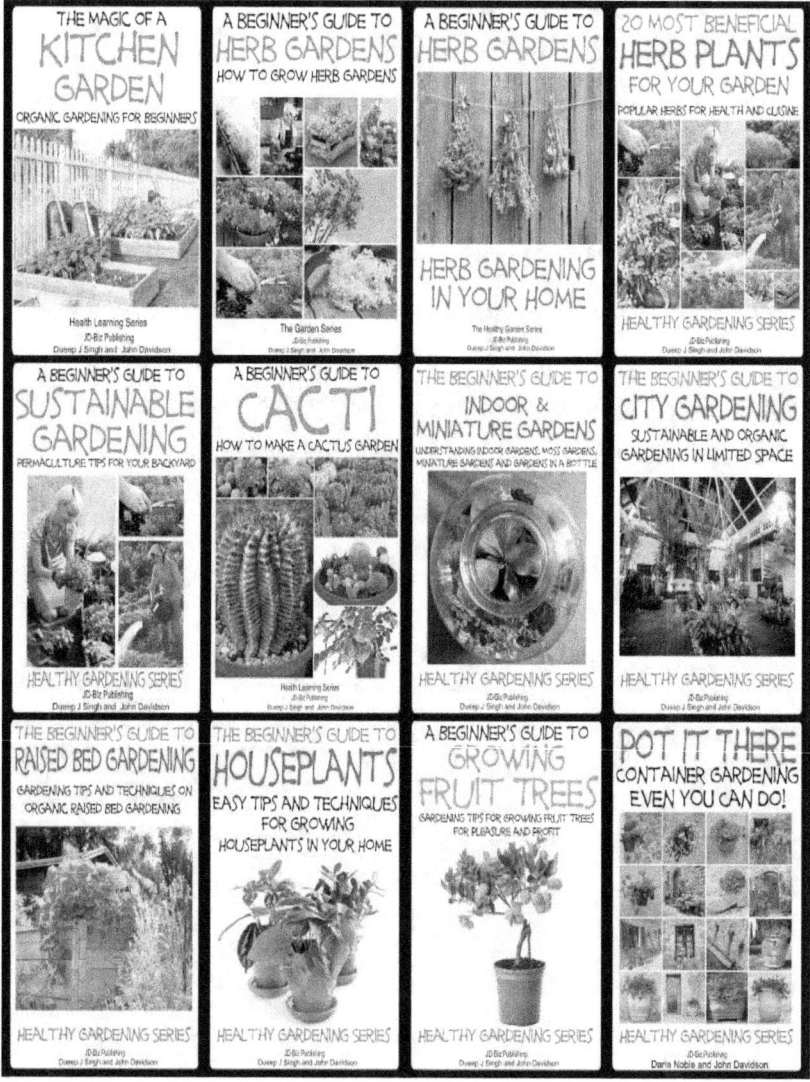

Health Learning Series

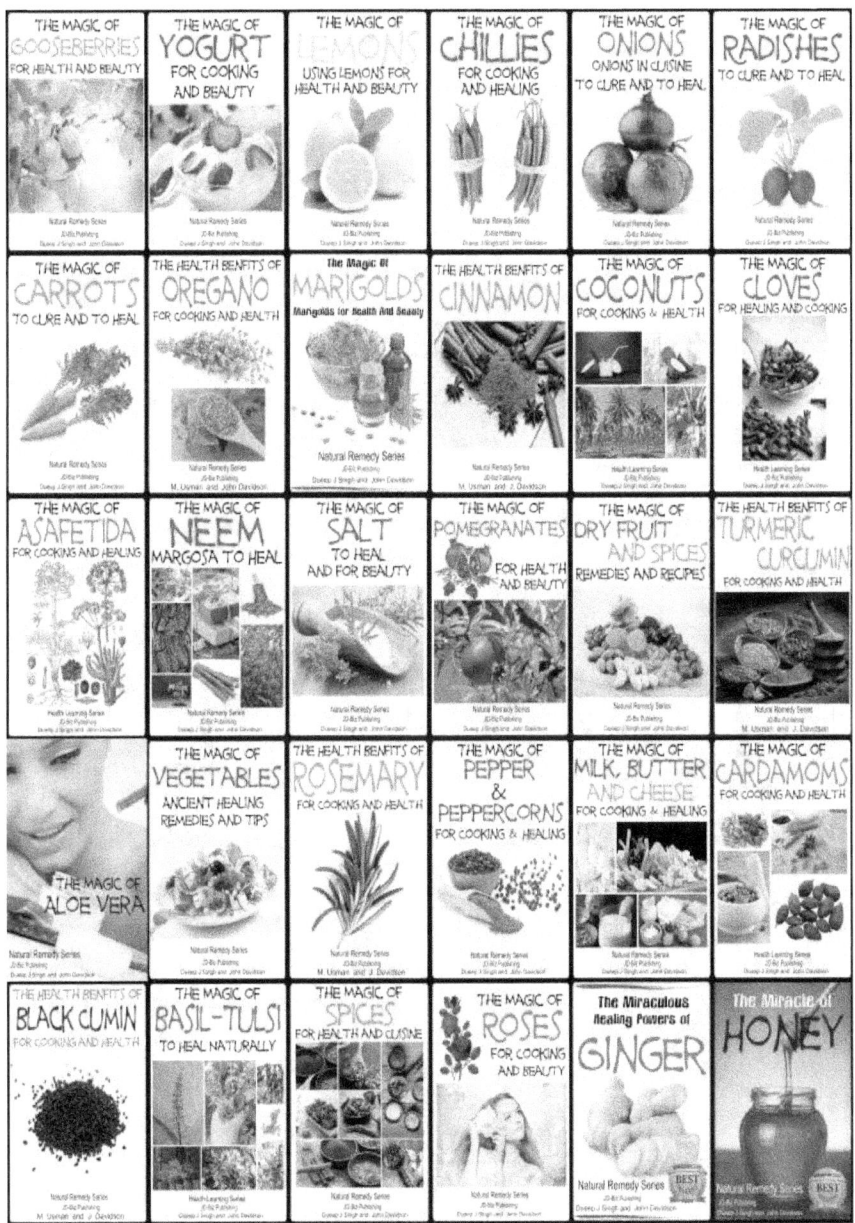

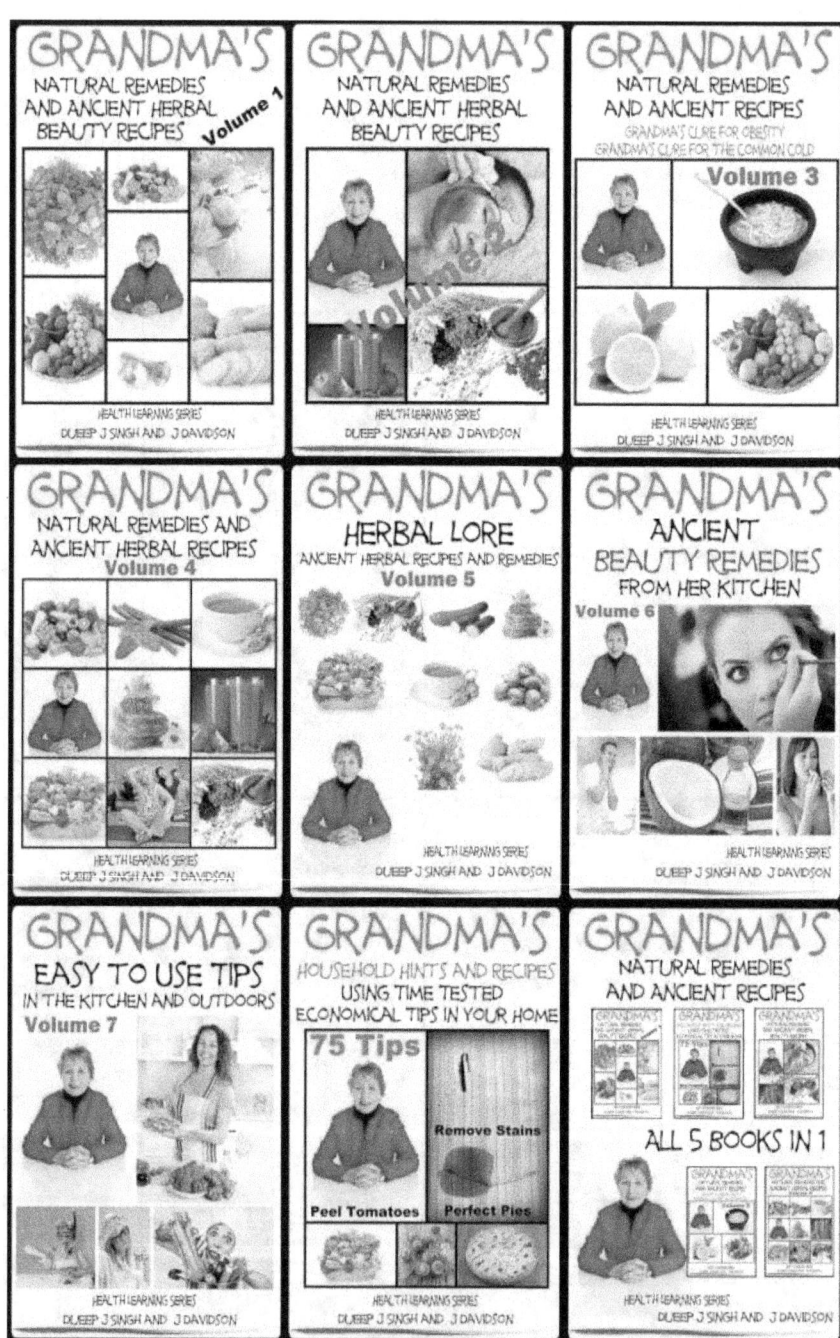

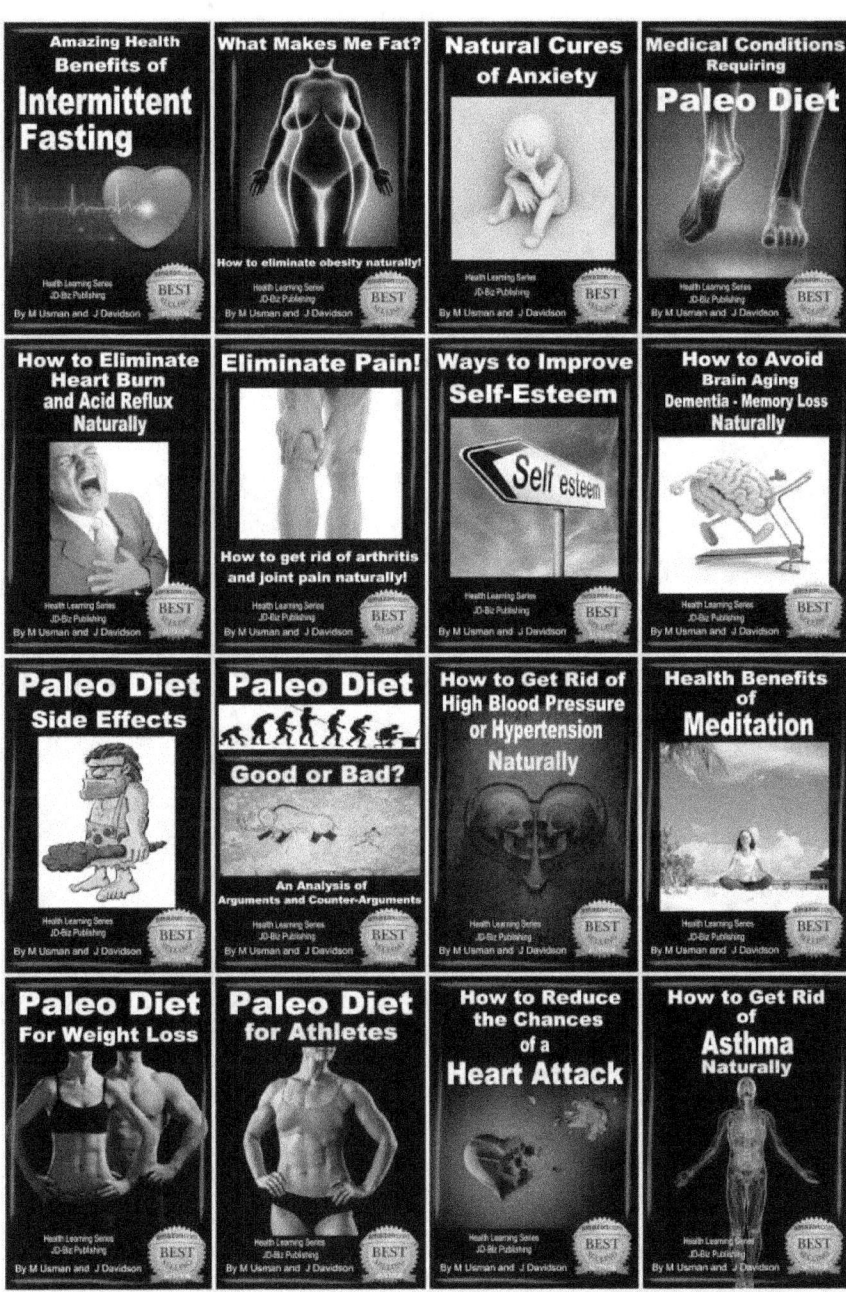

Amazing Animal Book Series

Learn To Draw Series

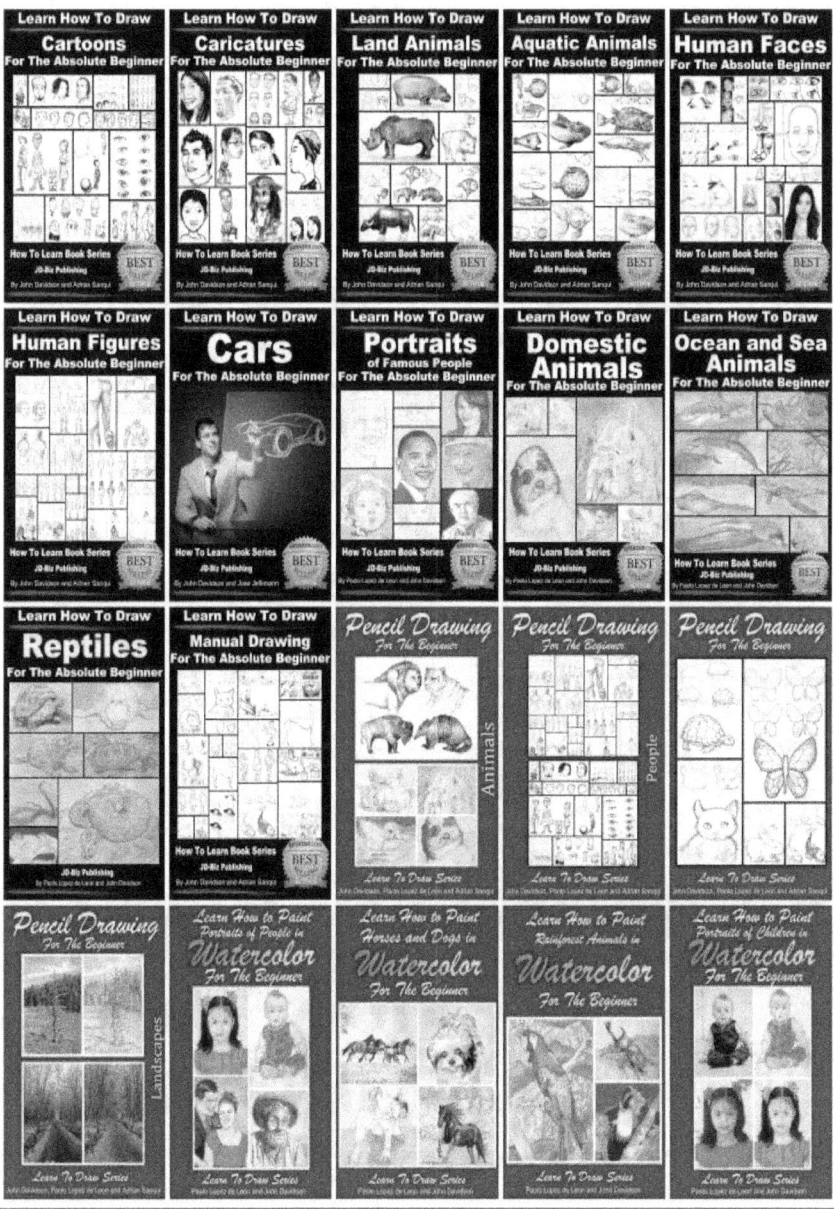

How to Build and Plan Books

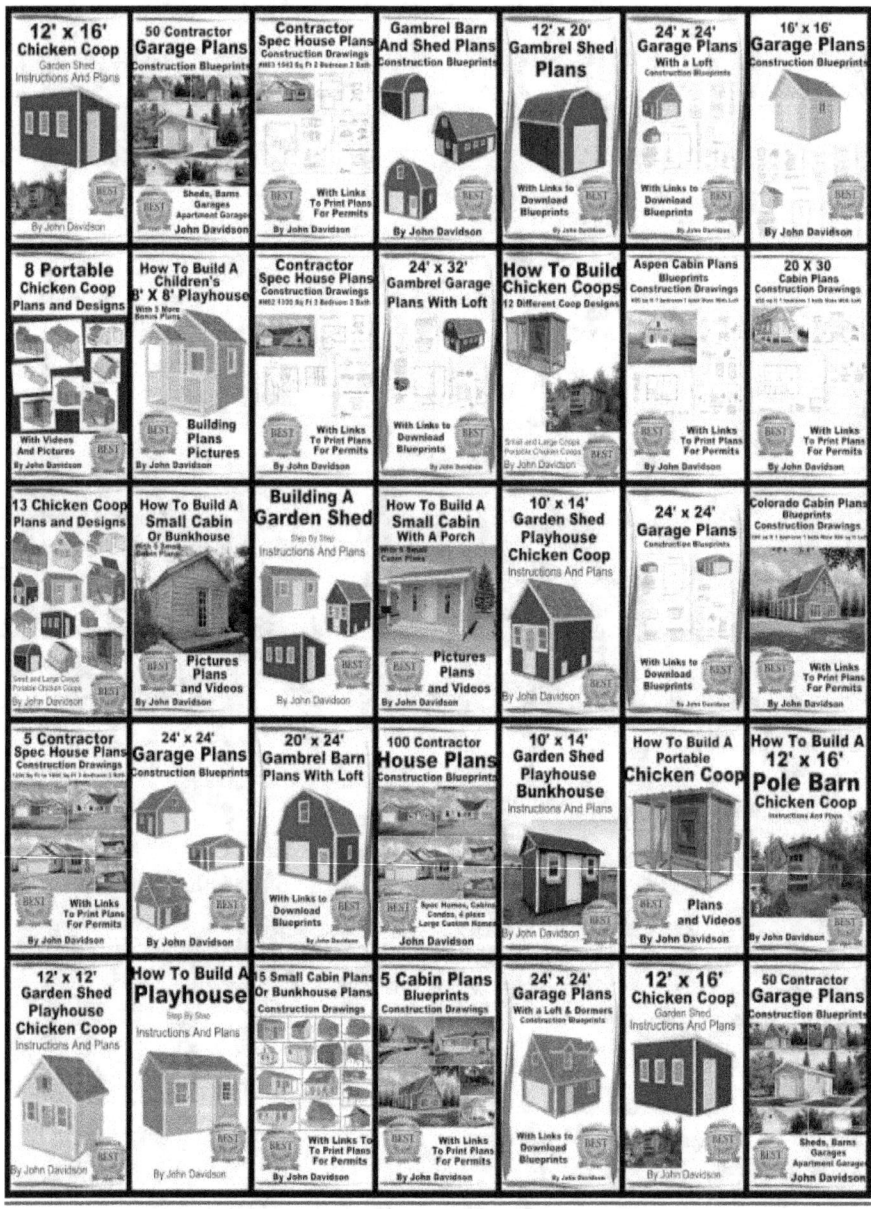

Entrepreneur Book Series

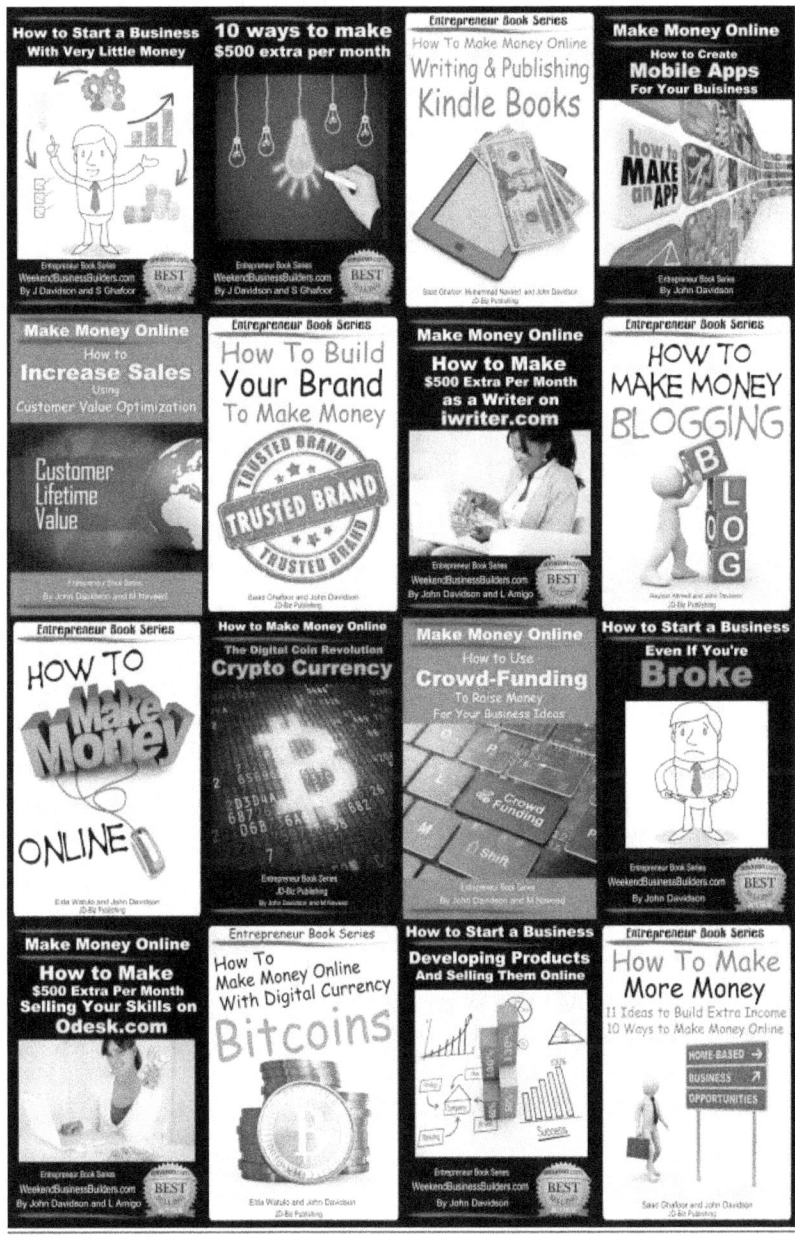

Our books are available at

1. Amazon.com

2. Barnes and Noble

3. Itunes

4. Kobo

5. Smashwords

6. Google Play Books

This book is published by

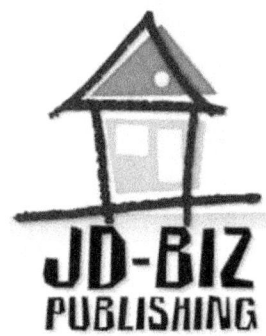

JD-Biz Corp

P O Box 374

Mendon, Utah 84325

http://www.jd-biz.com/

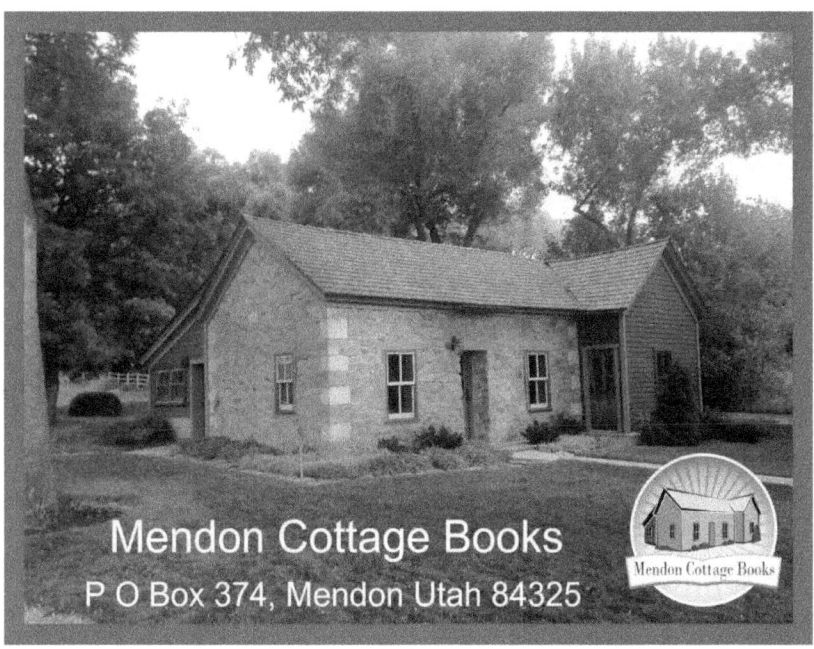

www.ingramcontent.com/pod-product-compliance
Lightning Source LLC
Chambersburg PA
CBHW071154280526
45787CB00003B/1505